Yasmin the Yoga Cat

Yasmin the Yoga Cat

Jean Romano

ReadersMagnet, LLC

Yasmin the Yoga Cat
Copyright © 2021 by Jean Romano

Published in the United States of America
ISBN Paperback: 978-1-955603-11-9
ISBN eBook: 978-1-955603-10-2

All rights reserved. No part of this publication may be reproduced, stored in a retrieval system or transmitted in any way by any means, electronic, mechanical, photocopy, recording or otherwise without the prior permission of the author except as provided by USA copyright law.

The opinions expressed by the author are not necessarily those of ReadersMagnet, LLC.

ReadersMagnet, LLC
10620 Treena Street, Suite 230 | San Diego, California, 92131 USA
1.619.354.2643 | www.readersmagnet.com

Book design copyright © 2021 by ReadersMagnet, LLC. All rights reserved.
Cover design by Ericka Obando
Interior design by Mary Mae Romero

INTRODUCTION

When children first attend school many adjustments are needed. Teachers are trained to help pre-schoolers and pre-readers find both an independent path to learning and the ability to become socially and emotionally adjusted to life in and out of the classroom. They do their job well. Those who have observed a pre-school class on the first day and again the last day of school are astonished by the change in behavior, self-confidence and skills.

In the first days, children find friendship, support, and independence. The years stretching from age four to eight are critical. Skills are important but becoming part of a community is even more so. Finding a common activity is one way of achieving this objective.

In a time of virtual learning, zoom classrooms, tablets and ipads; there has to be new ways of finding both self and social competence. It is suggested that meditation can be one path to these goals. It brings a child's focus on inner feelings that are shared with classmates. Although unique to each participant, it is the journey that brings children together. And the experience of allowing thoughts to float past the troubles of the day can give lasting benefits throughout a lifetime.

The physical exercise is designed to start with an activity that is fun. It allows for creative sharing by zoom or alone, and it does command attention. A child or a classroom following directions copies each yoga pose, modeled by a picture of a cat. There are no wrong answers. The activity can be extended by asking students to think of other ways to show how the pose could be demonstrated.

Part two of the opening routine is meditation. Explain that to a pre-schoolers? Of course! The child has been directed to move his or her body into different positions. Now the goal is to move the mind as well.

The five senses can be used to imagine past experiences. Eyes closed, body relaxed, thoughts free to explore. There are other directions related to mental health issues that can be helpful to young children. One is the Gratitude Journal. The simple closing of each day's routine can be linked to verbalizing something, someone, somewhere that makes the participant thankful.

This method of starting a particular learning objective for the daily curriculum does several services. It calms the child or classroom, provides a common experience, and allows for a release from immediate troubles or concerns. As Yasmin says, "there are no wrong answers". It is recommended for home schooling parents as well as trained teachers who now are faced with the problems unanticipated a short time ago.

MY NAME IS YASMIN

I am going to share some secrets with you.
My life is my own although always in view
of the family I live with by night and by day.
I'm here to help you. What more can I say?

I've written this very short guide
to teach you of actions you haven't yet tried.
Try to believe you can act like a cat
who hopes you will soon have your own yoga mat.

We will start with the physical actions required
to effectively reach all the true goals desired.
When your body can move into yoga positions
your mind will be ready to make new traditions.

All of the ways you can turn, bend, and twist
help you become a real Yoga artiste!
There are so many ways to arrange necks and noses
and each brings awareness of good yoga poses.

Let's begin with my favorite. I do this each morning.
If you're not a cat, take care, here's a warning.
If your legs don't return to a normal position
it's a sign that you didn't complete the transition
from four legged cat to more human ambition.

Soon you will see what I'm talking about.
It is simple for me and for you I've no doubt.
Forget any chores you've forgotten to do,
think only of putting each part somewhere new.

POSES AND DIRECTIONS

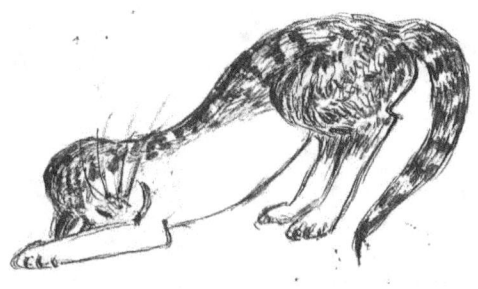

1. Praise

Lie on your stomach, head facing down and place hands in front of your head, flat on the floor. Slowly bring your knees forward and then raise your legs so they are straight and hip length apart. Hold this for three minutes or until you hear a clap!

2. Resting Left

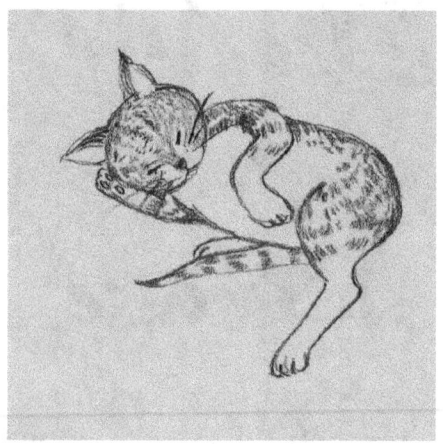

Lie on your left side. Bring left hand under your head. Raise left foot upwards until your knee touches your stomach. Place right hand on your stomach. Extend right leg out straight. Hold until clap.

3. Master Twist

Lie on your right side. Extend your right arm for balance. Bring head to left shoulder. Place left hand behind head. Extend left leg and pull right leg tow toward right hand. Hold until clap.

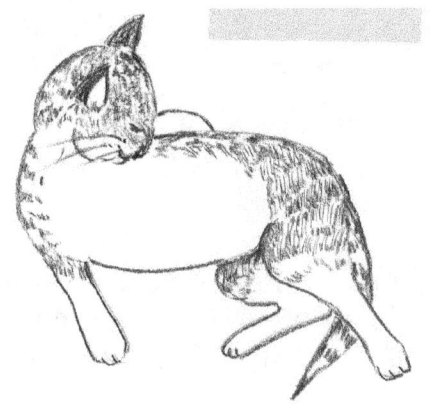

4. Pride

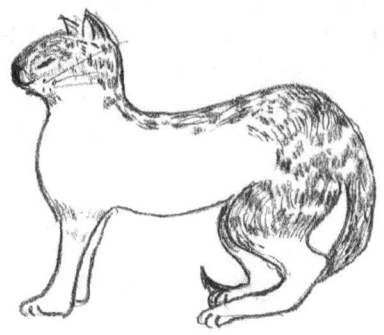

Stand straight and look straight ahead, head high. Hands straight down and feet straight and apart hips length. Don't smile! Hold!

5. Pouncing Cat

Stand straight. Bend elbow close to your body,
hands raised and facing outwards. Curve fingers
into claws. Bend knees far as you can. Hold!

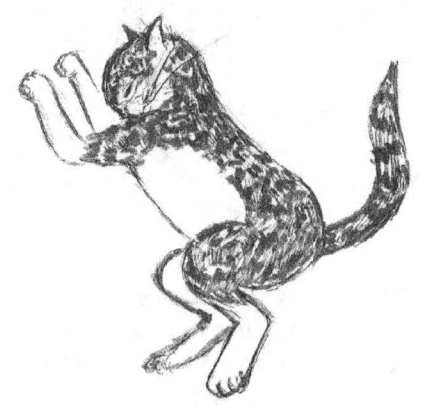

6. Relaxation

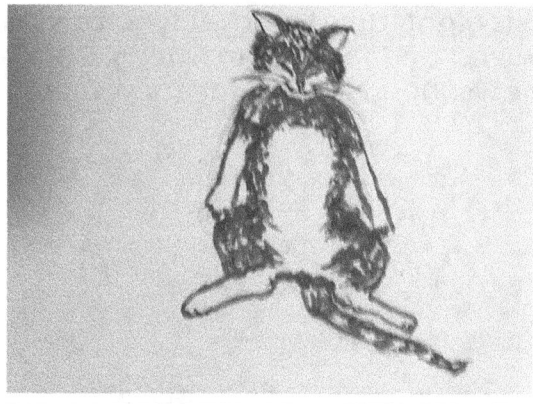

Lie on your back. Bend arms and let hands hang loosely on your chest. Draw knees close to stomach and then let them fall to your sides. Take deep breaths.

Don't try all these poses. Make some of your own.
Select those you like, don't cry and moan.
There's many a path to a fresh point of view
fashioned and practiced only by you.

We've covered so much active stuff!
You've done quite well but it's enough.
Together we move from physical to mental
and any new poses are just accidental.
There is only one body part you must control.
Close your eyes and you've done it! We're ready to roll.

I'm very clean and flexible because of my routine
from ears to toes I wash and screen
for fleas and ticks and things unseen.
This takes both dedication and a splash of
meditation.

I am sure you're amazed at the moves you can do.
Add a mental component and voila! Yoga Two!
Move from body to mind with wonderful ease.
I'll be your model. It will be a breeze!

My eyes are still open and what do I see?
A person ready to meditate with me.
The center of all my good advice
is meditation. Say it twice!

I appear to be sleeping but that isn't true.
I'm in full meditation and you will be too.
Can you guess what I'm hoping for?
You can't be wrong, I'll say no more.

If your eyes are closed, how can you see?
It's a matter of using your memory.
Do you remember your best friend's smile?
Just let it into your thoughts for awhile.
There are so many good things you can recall
like the sound of rustling leaves in the fall.
Let's try for something you can smell!
An apple covered with hot caramel,
A cake just taken from the oven,
fresh baked cookies by the dozen.

Keep on, keep on let's try one more.
Imagine stepping on a cold, cold floor
Or petting a cat. This one I adore.
Use your powers to think of good things
that take you to magical imaginings.

Here is my start but make a long list
of your special memories. I insist.
The sound of an acorn falling to the ground
Your breathing
The wind through the trees
Footsteps from far away
The crackle of a fireplace
Raindrops on the roof
Silence itself

SEE WITH CLOSED EYES

A friend's face
A special place
The door that welcomes you home
A path that leads you home
A favorite pet

FEEL

The sun on your face
Rain on your head
Water from an ocean wave
Your pet's fur
Your mother's hug
Each part of your body
One thing that made you happy today
A moment of joy

All these things are in your mind
Meditation's now defined.

MAKE ANOTHER LIST

WHAT IS HIDDEN IN YOUR MIND?

These are the five senses. Use them if you can.
Be grateful if you have all five, some do not and
must improvise. As you think about each sense, be
thankful for each as you commence!

I SEE
I HEAR
I FEEL
I TASTE
I SMELL

Ask why I practice this ancient art
beneficial to me and to you when you start.
Tell your body to let your mind
float in the air and put trouble behind.
Happy things are yours forever.
Remembering is your endeavor.

I leave you now but you can borrow
All my guidance for tomorrow.

POST SCRIPT AND REFERENCES

The children participating in this activity learn a technique that can last long past this period of distance learning and isolation. The practice of mindfulness and gratitude expression are life-long skills. It does become a routine.

Social-emotional issues are high on the list of priorities in education. They remain at the top of the list. It is time to expand on ways to address this concern. Many references to mental health are available on-line. One reference is especially timely and brings the fun of copying a cat to a more recognizable form. Best Yoga Poses for Kids- Pure Wow https://www.purewow.com/family/yoga-poses-for-kids

The National Association of School Psychologists offers a guide for teachers and parents to support children's mental health and their website is an excellent source for additional information. A specific article is cited below. Katherine C, Cowan, the author, is an asset to our times. National Association of School Psychologists (2017). Supporting children's mental health: Tips for parents and educators (Handout), Bethesda, MD: Author.

www.ingramcontent.com/pod-product-compliance
Lightning Source LLC
LaVergne TN
LVHW021051100526
838202LV00082B/5459